CLUB SWINGING

for Physical Exercise
and Recreation

A Book of Information About All Forms
of Indian Club Swinging Used in Gym-
nasiums and by Individuals

By

W. J. SCHATZ

With an Introduction by

W. G. ANDERSON, M. D.

Professor of Physical Education,
Yale University

———

Illustrated from Original Drawings

Exercises Progressively Arranged

———

American Gymnasia Company,
Boston, Mass., U. S. A.

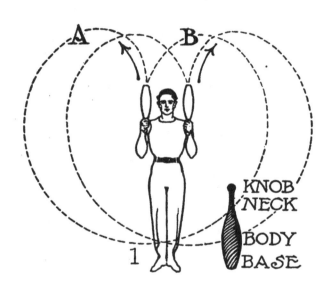

CONTENTS.

Contents.

Index to Illustrations on last page.

Windham Press is committed to bringing the lost cultural heritage of ages past into the 21st century through high-quality reproductions of original, classic printed works at affordable prices.

This book has been carefully crafted to utilize the original images of antique books rather than error-prone OCR text. This also preserves the work of the original typesetters of these classics, unknown craftsmen who laid out the text, often by hand, of each and every page you will read. Their subtle art involving judgment and interaction with the text is in many ways superior and more human than the mechanical methods utilized today, and gave each book a unique, hand-crafted feel in its text that connected the reader organically to the art of bindery and book-making.

We think these benefits are worth the occasional imperfection resulting from the age of these books at the time of scanning, and their vintage feel provides a connection to the past that goes beyond the mere words of the text.

As bibliophiles, we are always seeking perfection in our work, and so please notify us of any errors in this book by emailing us at corrections@windhampress.com. Our team is motivated to correct errors quickly so future customers are better served. Our mission is to raise the bar of quality for reprinted works by a focus on detail and quality over mass production.

To peruse our catalog of carefully curated classic works, please visit our online store at www.windhampress.com.

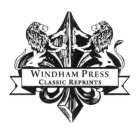

INTRODUCTION

By W. G. ANDERSON, M. D.

Professor of Physical Education, and
Director of Gymnasium, Yale University.

———————

AFTER a quarter of a century's experience teach-
ing gymnastics I feel more strongly drawn
than ever to the use of the clubs as a helpful and
pleasing form of exercise.

True, there are some objections to them from the
so-called hygienic standpoint, but these objections are
out-weighed by the factors in their favor. The ar-
guments against the club movements may just as
rightly be made against many of the movements
given with the wands and bells, but as it is possible
and probable that the exercises which bring the arms
too much in front of the body are at once counter-
acted by circles that raise the shoulders and draw
back the scapulae, I doubt much if any harm comes
pleasing form of exercise.

The time will never come I hope when the ele-
ment of pleasure in exercise will be overlooked.
There is more that is pleasurable in club swinging,
especially accompanied by good music, than in many

movements with other pieces of light apparatus and
I have noticed that pupils call for the clubs more fre-
quently than for bells or wands.

Only the most expert performer wil approximate
the mastery of the clubs; the combinations are so
numerous and difficult that one must be a specialist
to even stand on the threshold of complete knowledge of the thousand and one movements.

A limited use of the gray matter will enable one to
learn many movements without a teacher, especially
if he has a book like this at his elbow. The simple
circles made with wrist or arm either in front of or
back of the body above the head, at the shoulders or
waist to "reel," "follow" or "double" time, will open
a field for work that is very hard to cover.

When we further consider that every circle can be
reversed, that all snakes may be reversd, no matter
what the cadence or "time," and that the component
parts of the snakes may be used and also reversed,
we have before us a series of bewildering combinations that will call for years of work to learn.

As a remedial and curative agent in sprains and
strains of the shoulder, elbow and wrist points I have
had pronounced success with light clubs. Wrestlers,
foot and base-ball players, and gymnasts, have been
greatly aided in getting back the normal tonicity of
ligaments and muscles by "reels," wrist circles, etc.

That the Indian Club is the only piece of light apparatus adopted by the collegiate and intercollegi-

9

ate gymnastic societies is an argument in its favor not to be lightly passed by.

As physical training is constantly progressive there is a field for any book that is thoroughly up to date. I have examined Mr. Schatz's work and find it good.

Mr. Schatz is an expert club swinger as well as a teacher of gymnastics, hence he can and has combined the knowledge of the former with the experience of the latter in such a manner as to produce a book that will be helpful alike to teacher and pupil.

W. G. ANDERSON.

Part I.

ELEMENTARY CLUB SWINGING.

PART I.

ELEMENTARY CLUB SWINGING.

The *proper starting position* is shown in Fig. 1. Stand erect, chest arched, heels about two inches apart, and feet at an angle of forty-five degrees. Look straight ahead, don't move the body unless so directed; let the arm do the swinging, or rather let the club swing the arm. The body should remain as motionless as a statue; the arms should act as moving appendages. Little effort is required to keep the club in motion, for after it is started its own weight will almost do the work.

The *grasp* of the club varies with the different work to be done, but the club is generally held between the thumb and first two fingers. If the club is held with the thumb and all the fingers, some movements cannot be executed which the above grasp renders easy. The grasp with its variations will be explained from time to time as occasion requires. For the benefit of the pupil, special pains were taken in order to secure accurate illustrations of the grasp and the positions.

Circles,—arm and hand. An *arm circle* is a circle made by swinging the club with the arm extended, the shoulder being the center of the circle. The term *arm circle* is generally used to denote any part of a circle described by extending the arm as in Fig. 1 from "a" to "b;" and the term *full-arm circle* is used to designate a complete circle described with the club.

A *hand circle*, sometimes called the *short or wrist* circle, is made by describing a circle with the base of the club, the hand being the center of the circle. (Fig. 4.)

A *heart-shaped circle* is shown in Fig. 1.

A *pendulum* is usually an arm circle going from shoulder high to shoulder high, but the arc described may be more or less than a half-circle.

Directions: Circles are executed right and left, forward and backward, in the vertical plane, and right and left in the horizontal plane; in fact they may be executed in almost any conceivable plane and direction.

It will be noticed that in this work few circles are described that are not executed to the right and left, that is, in a vertical plane parallel to a plane passing from side to side through the body, when standing at *attention;* the reason being that the effect of forward and backward movements can easily be reached by simply turning the trunk to the right or left. At the same time the continuous motion of the club, thus swung, contributes to the ease of learning combinations and exercises, which, if the club were swung in mixed planes, would be more confusing. This method is also more effective in exhibition work, as it presents a better view to the spectator.

All circles are considered as starting from the starting position, and are named accordingly.

When a circle is started away from the head, by swinging the club in the lateral plane, that is, the right club to the right, the left club to the left, it is called an *outward circle;* when toward the head an *inward*

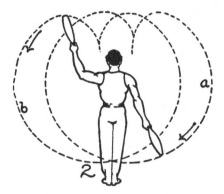

circle. Fig. 1 shows a *double outward circle.* In swinging in the other planes the circles are named from the direction the club takes when it starts the circle, as *backward, forward,* etc. These latter movements are given in Part IV.

The Pendulum movements, etc., where the club is swung in one direction, then brought to a stop, then swung with the direction reversed, have been left for Part IV, because it has been thought best to give the continuous movements first. It is hoped that this method will be helpful to the pupil, as a pupil who swings an arm circle will often hesitate before doing the hand circle, supposed to follow it, because he does not know which direction the club is to go. For this reason the continuous movements have been arranged together, and all the pupil will have to do is to allow the club to swing in the direction it naturally will take, thereby indicating its proper course. It will be seen that one of the first requisites, then, is to hold the club easily, and to swing it with just enough effort to keep it going, and merely direct it. This applies especially to fancy work.

The work contained in this volume has been arranged in progressive order, and the transition from the very simple to the most intricate work has been as gradual as could be conveniently planned. Some of the movements can be very easily acquired, though others will require perseverance and long practice to master.

Always practice the movement first with one hand; then, after the movement is mastered with that hand, take the other; and finally use both together. Practice each movement until it becomes almost automatic, so that the movement is thought of simply while the club moves along smoothly with scarcely any conscious effort on the part of the performer.

Standing in front of a mirror in very helpful to the pupil, as it gives him an exact idea of how he is performing.

LESSON I.

HEART-SHAPED CIRCLES.

1. From starting position, raise the right club upward and outward, extending the arm; as you reach "a" (Fig. 1), let the club swing as indicated, coming to position again. This is an *outward heart-shaped circle*.

2. Continue the movement a number of times, and as the club swings from that part of the arc marked "a" to "b," count 1; and as the club is brought down to position, count 2; let there be a little bound to the movement from "b" to "a." (This bound will help later when the hand circle is substituted for count 2.) In the heart-shaped circle the circle is 1, and the bound 2; in the regular work it would be 1 for the arm circle and 2 for the hand circle.

3. Same as exercise 2, but use the left.

4. Swing both clubs outward simultaneously, describing a heart-shaped circle with each hand. This is a *double outward heart-shaped circle*. (Circle 1, bound 2). Fig. 1 shows this exercise.

5. Swing club inward, executing a right *inward heart-shaped circle*. Repeat for left.

6. *Double inward heart-shaped circle*. In exercises 5 and 6, the clubs move in a direction opposite to that indicated in Fig. 1.

17

7. Swing right outward circle 1, bound 2; then swing left outward circle 3, bound 4; continue for 16 counts.

8. Swing right outward circle 1, bound 2; and have left start an outward while the right is executing count 1; the left executing the bound on 1 and circle on 2. Fig. 2 shows position of right club when the left is starting.

9. Same as exercise 7, but inward.

10. Same as exercise 8, but inward.

11. Starting both clubs together, swing a left inward and a right outward heart-shaped circle. Fig. 3 shows the start; and, at X, the relative position of the clubs as they swing downward. They remain parallel throughout the entire movement. Circle, count 1; bound, count 2. This is known as the *parallel movement.*

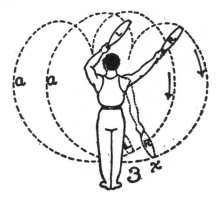

LESSON II.

HAND CIRCLES.

1. Hold the club in front of the body as in Fig 4; let it fall forward, continuing the circle as indicated. This is a *forward hand circle;* also known as an *outward hand circle in front.* Circle for 16 counts.

2. (A) Start as above, but with both hands held in front of body and executing forward circles; (B) gradually separate hands, bringing them backward until they are at sides. In this movement the clubs execute outward circles;—*double forward hand circles* in A, and *double outward hand circles* in B. The latter is generally called a *shoulder circle* instead of a *hand circle.* Fig. 5 shows the right hand executing an outward shoulder circle.

3. Same as exercise 1; but let club fall backward toward shoulder, and continue the circle for 16 counts. This is a *backward circle in front,* or as sometimes called, an *inward circle in front,* because the club falls inward toward the shoulder.

4. Same as exercise 2; but circle backward. In this movement the club will come to the sides swinging the *double inward shoulder circle.*

LESSON III.

ARM AND SHOULDER CIRCLES.

1. As in Lesson I, exercise 2, start right arm circle outward, count 1; but for count 2, instead of the bound, substitute a shoulder circle outward. Repeat for left.

2. Same as exercise 1, but inward.

3. Same as exercise 1, but double outward; also double inward.

4. Parallel arm and shoulder circles to the right, that is, same as Lesson I, exercise 11; but substitute shoulder circles for count 2.

In order to render this parallel movement less difficult to learn, let the pupils start heart-shaped circles to the right as in Lesson I, exercise 11; but instead of starting from position, lay clubs on the shoulders, with the trunk turned to the right, and swing the clubs parallel upward and to the right. As the clubs come downward to execute the arm circle, turn the trunk front, 1; then, as the clubs rise on the left side, turn trunk left and receive clubs on shoulders; then turn trunk to the right and start again, 2. Continue this movement; but gradually lay the clubs farther back at every circle,, until they finally hang down the back. By so doing, the pupil will find himself executing the

20

full *parallel movement* with *arm and shoulder circles.* Of course, after the movement is learned, the pupil must gradually diminish the trunk-turning until the movement is done with trunk front during the entire exercise.

In this movement great care should be exercised that the shoulder circles are started at exactly the same time, so that the movements will be truly parallel.

5. Execute two outward shoulder circles with the right, 1 and 2; at same time swing left arm circle outward, 1, and left shoulder circle, 2; continue for 16 counts.

6. Same as exercise 5, but execute the continuous shoulder circles with the left, and the arm and shoulder circle with the right.

7. Swing double outward shoulder and arm circles as in exercise 3. After swinging continuously for 8 counts, instead of executing an arm and shoulder circle with the right, substitute two shoulder circles, and then proceed as before with the arm and shoulder circle. The movement executed is an *alternate movement;* that is, a right shoulder circle and a left arm circle simultaneously, and a right arm circle and a left shoulder circle simultaneously. This movement is known as the *reel.*

8. To change from the alternate movement to the *double movement,* substitute two shoulder circles for the arm and shoulder circles made by the right.

9. The *follow movement,* or *windmill.* In this movement, going to the right, the right executes an outward shoulder circle, 4; and an arm circle outward, 2; the left executes an inward shoulder circle, 3, and an arm circle, 1; the clubs are a quarter circle apart at all times during the movement. Fig. 6 shows this movement.

This movement is sometimes difficult to learn, but if the following method is used it can be mastered quite readily. Start parallel movement as in exercise 4; after 4 counts, as soon as the shoulder circles have been executed, instead of having clubs come down into parallel arm circle, let the left lead a little; increase this lead at every circle until the clubs are just a quarter circle apart.

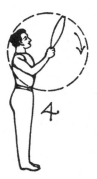 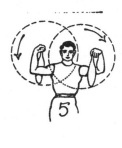

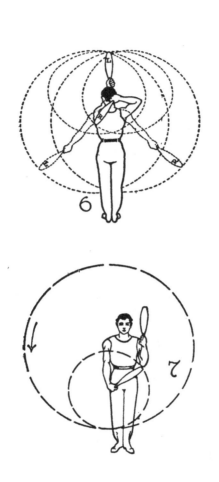

6

7

LESSON IV.

COMBINATIONS OF HAND AND ARM CIRCLES.

There are a great variety of hand circles to be combined with arm circles,—a list of those most used follows. Practice each separately with each hand, inward and outward, and combine each with an arm circle. Fig. 5 shows the right executing a shoulder circle and the left and upper front. These circles are sometimes executed with the arms more nearly extended than shown in the illustration. The shoulder circle is executed with the *ring grip*, the club rolling around loosely in the ring formed by the thumb and forefinger. Fig. 46 shows plainly the ring grip on the right hand, as do Figs. 6, 11 and 12.

The *upper front circle* is executed with the hand and the handle of club forming a *ball and socket* joint; (Fig. 5). The wrist is not flexed in this circle; but the handle of the club, held by thumb and forefinger, rolls around loosely in the grasp, thus forming the assumed ball-and-socket joint.

1. Continuous upper fronts with right, same with left; same double. Practice them in both outward and inward movements.

2. Continuous shoulder circles with right; same with left; same double. Inward and outward movements.

3. Upper front outward with right, 1; arm circle outward, 2. Same left. Same double.

4. Same as exercise 3, but inward movement.

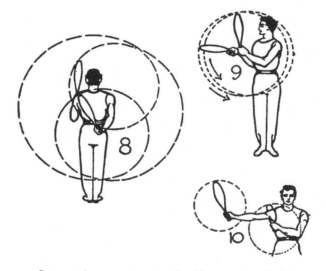

5. Outward movement, double arm circle, 1; double upper front, 2; double shoulder, 3.

6. Same, inward movement.

7. Same, parallel movement, right and left.

8. Right executes shoulder circle, 1, and upper front, 2, while left executes the upper front, 1, and

shoulder circle, 2. This movement is known as the *short reel*.

9. Change from reel to short reel, to reel, etc.

The *lower front circle*. Fig. 7 shows lower front outward combined with arm circle. The lower front is executed with the ring grip.

10. Continuous lower fronts, inward movement, each hand; also outward movement. Each 16 counts.

11. Combine arm circle and lower front, outward movement, with the right, for 16 counts; (Fig. 7). Same inward.

12. Outward movements; combine arm circle, 1, lower front, 2, and upper front, 3; continue for 12 counts. Same inward. Each hand separately.

13. Combine right outward upper front, 1, shoulder 2, arm, 3, and lower front, 4. Same inward. Same left.

It will be noticed that when combinations are executed in which the lower front is used it appears to count two; this happens because on coming down from position to lower front only one-half of the arm circle is executed, and the other half is executed after the lower front has been completed. The first count, 1, is really the first half of the arm circle and the first half of the lower front; and the second count, 2, is the second half of the lower front and the second half of the arm circle.

14. Execute exercises 11, 12, and 13 double.

The *lower back outward*. Take a firm grip on club

and start from position; swing outward and downward and back of hip, and, as the club rises, bend the wrist; as club rises to position occupied by club in Fig. 8, which shows right executing lower front, draw the hand forward, keeping it close to the body. In the inward movement the hand is held close to the body while the club is going back, instead of close to body on coming forward. Practice inward and outward combined, with the arm circle, each hand separately.

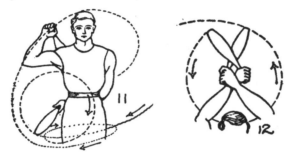

The *extended arm, hand circle*. Fig. 10 shows the right executing this circle. It is generally executed with arm horizontal, obliquely upward and obliquely downward. The circle is executed both in front of and in back of the arm.

Under Arm Circle. Fig. 10 shows left executing the under arm; dotted line shows course of club behind body.

Over Arm Circle. Fig. 16 shows the left executing

27

the over arm inward. Fig. 14 shows right executing an outward over arm circle. The word "arm-circle" is used to denote the act of making an arm circle or part thereof.

Waist Circles are four in number. In Fig. 11 the left is executing a *front waist, arm over back*. If the left in this position were to execute a circle behind the body, it would be doing a *back waist, arm over back*. If, as in Fig. 10, the left were brought down waist high and the circle executed behind the body, it would be a *back waist, arm over front;* and if the circle were executed in front of the body, it would be a *front waist, arm over front*.

After the hand circles given thus far have been practiced with each hand separately, they can be combined with arm circles, both inward and outward, in the parallel, follow, and in the double and alternate movements. Examples follow in lessons on advanced work.

In the preceding lessons the elementary work has been given. The work that follows consists of combinations of these elements, with the addition of the snakes and spirals. As nearly as is consistent, the work follows in graded form.

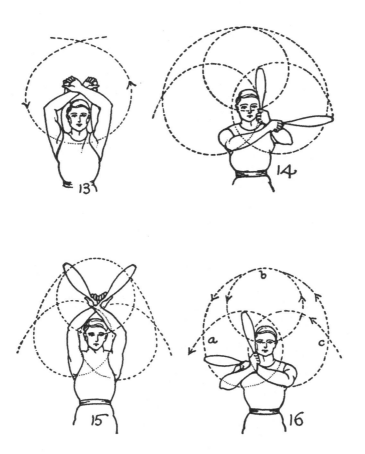

Part II.

ADVANCED CLUB SWINGING.

PART II

ADVANCED CLUB SWINGING

LESSON I

SHOULDER CIRCLES.

1. Double shoulder circle, 1, double arm circle, 2; outward or inward movement.

2. Alternate movement, left shoulder circle and right arm circle, 1, right shoulder circle and left arm circle, 2; outward or inward.

3. Execute two shoulder circles, right outward, 1, 2, arm circle to lower front and up again, 3, 4. This combination is sometimes known as the *long reel*. Same inward movement.

4. Double upper front circle, 1, double arm circle, 2; outward or inward movement.

5. Double upper front circle, 1, double arm circle to double lower front and up again, 2, 3; outward or inward movement.

6. Combine shoulder, upper front, and lower front in double movement, either inward or outward.

7. To exercise 6, add lower back circle.

8. Upper front, 1, shoulder, 2, arm extended horizontally, 3, arm extended obliquely downward, 4, lower back, 5, lower front, 6 and 7, shoulder, 8. Swing the above in the double outward movement.

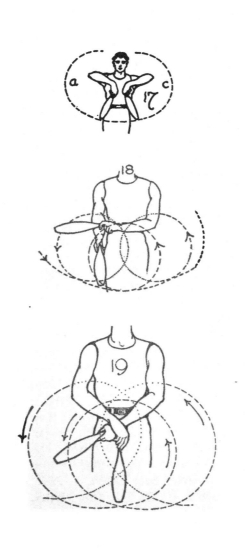

9. Double inward movement, arm circle down and lower front, 1, 2, hand circle, arm extended horizontally, 3, upper front, 4.

10. Change from the alternate movement into the double movement by substituting a hand circle for one of the arm circles with one hand. Change from double into alternate by the same method. If this change is made continuous, and once with right and then with left, a pleasing movement is the result.

11. Execute the long reel inward, and have the centers of the lower fronts and the shoulder circles directly in the median line of the body. Instead of the shoulder circles this becomes more of an extended arm hand circle above the head.

12. Alternate movement, two shoulder circles and lower back; outward movement.

13. Alternate movement, upper front, shoulder, and lower back; outward movement.

14. Alternate movement, upper front, shoulder circle, lower back and lower front; outward movement.

Observe that in the last three exercises the lower circles are made with one hand and the upper circles are extended with the other. The circles are executed with each hand in the order in which they are named.

15. Alternate movement; right executes shoulder circle, 2; trunk turning right; right executes a forward circle, 2; trunk turns forward and then to left as right is arm-circled over to left, 3, there executing a backward circle, 4; the left arm circles, 1, over to

34

right side as the trunk is turned to right and there describes a backward circle, 2; then as the trunk is turned front the left is swung up overhead and executes a forward circle, 4. To sum up, the left is executing an arm circle while the right is executing a shoulder circle; both hands are executing a circle in front of the body with the trunk turned to the right, the clubs are going in opposite directions; then, as the

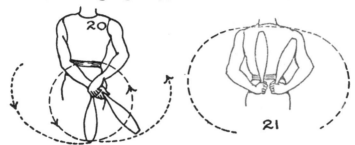

trunk is turned to the left, the left executes a shoulder circle and the right an arm circle, both meeting again in front of the body, each going in opposite directions; outward movement.

16. Same as above, except that an upper front is executed before the shoulder circle, and a lower back and lower front is added. The right executes upper front, 1; shoulder circle, 2; forward circle with trunk turned to right, 3; trunk turned front lower back, 4, and lower front, 5; backward circle with trunk turned to left, 6, the backward circle being made in this instance on the inside instead of on the outside of the

arm. The left executes a lower back, 1; lower front, 2; trunk turned to right, a backward circle on the inside of the arm, 3; trunk turned front upper front, 4; shoulder circle, 5; and trunk turned left a forward circle, 6, outward movement.

17. Start outward arm circle with both clubs; let left swing as in Fig. 11 to execute a front waist arm-over-back circle, while right makes an arm circle and also executes a shoulder circle, 1, 2; left comes out as in Fig. 11, swings up, and executes its shoulder circle, while the right executes two shoulder circles, 3, 4.

18. Let the right hand follow the work given to the left in exercise 17; and let the left execute the arm circle and three shoulder circles.

19. Combine the right work of exercise 18 with the left of exercise 17.

20. From position, arm-circle outward with both clubs, bringing them up as though to execute shoulder circles, but overlapping them as in Fig. 12 (the broken line and arrows indicate the course taken by left club). Let the clubs swing on, completing the hand circles, and be ready to go into arm circles.

Fig. 13 shows the position of the hands just before clubs rise again. The broken line and arrows indicate the course the left club has taken from the time the club rose overhead and executed its hand circle to the point where it is about to start another arm circle. This movement is known as the *scissors*.

LESSON II

PARALLEL CIRCLES

The movements are here described as going parallel to the right; naturally, the pupil should practice them to the left also. If the method given in Part I, Lesson III, Exercise 4, is employed in learning some of the movements here given, it will be easier to master the work; but as soon as they can be executed fairly well, perfect form should be observed. The body must remain like a statue, and the arms alone move. Sometimes the trunk is turned, and such exceptions are stated.

1. Parallel shoulder circles, 1, arm circles, 2.

2. Parallel upper fronts, 1, shoulder circles, 2, arm circles, 3.

3. Parallel upper fronts, 1, shoulder circles, 2, arm circles with lower front, 3, 4.

4. Parallel upper fronts, 1, shoulder circles, 2, arm circles with lower backs, 3, 4.

5. Parallel shoulder circles, 1, upper fronts, 2, shoulder circles, 3, arm circles with lower backs and and lower fronts, 4, 5, 6.

6. Continuous parallel upper fronts and shoulder circles, then arm-circle down and execute continuous lower backs and lower fronts, arm circles up again, etc.

7. Parallel upper fronts, 1, arm-circle with lower fronts, 2, 3.

8. Parallel shoulder circles, 1, arm-circle with lower backs, 2, 3.

9. Parallel upper fronts, 1, shoulder circles, 2, turning trunk to right, execute forward circles, 3; turning trunk forward again, lower backs and lower fronts, 4, 5 and 6; turning trunk left, execute backward circles, 7; turning trunk forward, execute shoulder circles, 8.

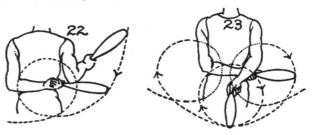

10. Same as above exercise; but on count 3 execute the forward circles with the arms crossed; that is, just as the shoulder circles have been executed and the trunk is turning to the right, cross arms, left wrist over right. The forward circles will be executed thus: the one with the right will be on outside of left forearm, the one with the left outside of right forearm; for count 7 execute the backward circles with arms crossed, left wrist on right wrist.

11. Execute with the right a lower back and a lower front, 1, 2, 3; execute with the left a lower front

and a lower back, 1, 2, 3; combine the right and left hand work and the *shift* is the result. This is sometimes called the *split* also.

12. Same as exercise 10, but substitute the *shift* for counts 4, 5, and 6.

13. Parallel, starting from position, arm circles, 1, right-over-arm circle and left-extended-horizontal hand circle, 2.

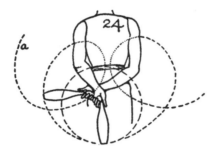

14. Parallel, starting from position, arm circles, 1, left-over-arm and right-extending horizontal, hand circle, 2.

15. Parallel arm circles, 1, shoulder and hand circles, as in exercise 13, 2, arm circles, 3, shoulder and hand circles, as in exercise 14, 4.

16. Same as exercise 15, but substitute upper fronts for count 3. The *parallel fountain* is the result.

17. Same as exercise 16, but for the arm circles, count 1, substitute a parallel short arm circle; Fig. 17 shows how the clubs are passed in this exercise.

18. Same as exercise 12, but for counts 1, 2, and 3 substitute right-over-arm and left-extended-horizontal hand circles, upper fronts, 2, and left-over-arm and right-extended-horizontal hand circles, 3.

19. Parallel movement; right-over-arm and left-extended-horizontal circles, 1; upper fronts, 2; left-over-arm and right-extended-horizontal, 3; left-under-arm and right-extended-horizontal hand circle (Fig. 10), 4; pass left around to execute a front waist arm-over back circle and at the same time circle right-extended-horizontal, 5; now execute the front waist arm-over-back circle and another circle right-extended-horizontal, 6; after having completed the waist circle swing the left over to the left-extended-horizontal position and the right to front waist arm-over-back position, 7; execute one circle here with each hand, 8; left-extended-horizontal circle and swing right around ready to execute an under-arm, 9; execute the right-under-arm circle and at the same time a left-extended-horizontal hand circle, 10; and the entire circuit has been made. Repeat the exercise four times.

On counts 6 and 8, the extended-arm-horizontal hand circle should be made in front of the arm instead of back of the arm, as, executed in this way, it will harmonize better, as the waist circles arm-over-back are fronts.

20. Parallel movement: arm circles, 1, shoulder circles, 2, left shoulder circle and right arm circle, 3, shoulder circles, 4.

PART TWO

21.   As in exercise 20, execute counts 1, 2, 3 and 4, but arm-circle left and shoulder circle right for 5, shoulder circles both right and left for 6; continue the exercise by continually repeating counts 3, 4, 5, and 6.

22.   This exercise as stated in exercise 21 may also be executed by continuing 3 and 5, but this is not so rhythmical, nor does it appear quite so pleasing to the eye.

23.   Left executes three shoulder circles while the right arm circles with a lower front and then shoulder-circles, 1, 2, 3; then the right executes there shoulder circles, while the left arm circles with a lower front and shoulder-circles again, 4, 5, 6.

24.   Same as the above exercise, but substitute lower backs instead of the lower fronts.

25.   Same as exercise 23, but execute four shoulder circles above and add a lower back below.

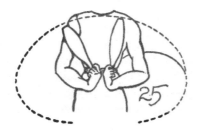

LESSON III

FOLLOW CIRCLES

The movements are described as going to the right. Naturally the pupil should practice them to the left also. The trunk turning principle may be employed here as in the parallels; but after the movement is learned, correct form should be observed.

1. Follow, left arm circle, 1, right arm circle, 2, left shoulder circle, 3, and right shoulder circle, 4.

2. Same as exercise 1, except that left executes an over arm circle on 3.

3. Same as exercise 1, except that right executes an over arm circle on 4.

4. Execute exercises 2 and 3 alternately.

5. Follow, left arm circle, 1, right arm circle, 2, left shoulder circle, 3, right over arm circle, 4, left upper front circle, 5, right upper front, 6, left over arm, 7, right shoulder circle 8. This movement, without counts 1 and 2, is known as the *upper fountain*. Fig. 14 shows how the clubs and hands are placed when about to execute counts 3 and 4; Fig. 15 shows position of clubs and arms starting to execute upper fronts. The pupil should be sure to have these circles well up. Fig. 16 shows the position of the clubs and hands when about to execute counts 7 and

42

8. The broken lines and arrows in the three figures indicate the course taken by the left club; "c" is the completed shoulder circle, "b" is the upper front, and "a" the over arm. The circles behind the shoulders should be executed well down; then the clubs should run up in executing the upper fronts; and then again come down to execute the circles behind.

6. Same as exercise 5, but instead of an arm circle pass clubs across chest by short arm circles, as is shown in Fig. 17. The line and arrows indicate course of right club; "a" is where the shoulder circle was completed and the short arm circle begun; "c" marks the place where the short arm ends and the over arm begins.

7. Left upper front circle, 1; right upper front, 2; left shoulder circle, 3; right shoulder circle, 4. After the exercise has been mastered as stated above, begin to straighten the arms while executing the shoulder circles, and try to keep the hands close together and directly above head.

8. Start an upper fountain, and as clubs come to the upper fronts introduce the continuous circles as given in exercise 7, executing them four times before completing the fountain. In all fountain movements it should be the aim to keep the hands close together; and, as in Fig. 14, the center of the over arm circle and shoulder circle should be exactly in the same place. The center of both the upper fronts should be exactly the same point, directly upward from the

43

median line of the head and about as nearly at arm's length as possible. The over arm and shoulder circles, also (see Fig. 15) should have their center as nearly as possible at the same point, which should be close to the body.

9. Follow arm circles, 1, 2; shoulder circles, 3, 4; forward follow circles, turning trunk to right, 5, 6; arm circle, trunk front, 7, 8; backward circles, turning trunk to left, 9, 10. Repeat, omitting arm circles, 1, 2. Fig. 9 shows follow circles forward, with trunk turned to left.

10. Execute the upper fountain, 1, 2, 3, 4, 5, 6; forward follows trunk turned to right, 7, 8; arm circles, 9, 10; backward follows trunk turned to left, 11, 12; continue. The forward circles at right, and backward circles at left, may be continued from four to six counts before proceeding to next movement.

11. See Lesson II, exercise 11, and practice it in the follow time. This is the *follow shift,* counting 1, 2, 3, 4, 5, 6.

12. Same as exercise 10, but for the arm circles 9 and 10 substitute the follow shift; which will give the entire movement 16 counts.

13. Same as exercise 11; but as the right comes behind the body to execute the lower back circle, place the wrist in the median line of the body and about waist high, and make a continuous lower back circle. The wrist thus pressed against the back will aid in

keeping the center of the continuous circles at the same place; meanwhile the left executes lower fronts, with center also in the median line in front and at the same level as that with which the lower backs are executed. After several continuous circles have been executed in this position, bring the right forward and execute continuous lower fronts, and bring the left back, executing continuous lower backs; the same rule as to the centers of the circles in the median line of body, and same level also, in the median line of bodys, and same level also, applies here.

This movement is known, on account of the resemblance, as the *pin wheel*. With decorated clubs, it has the fullest effect. Care must be taken that the movement is executed in strict follow time.

LESSON IV

FOLLOW CIRCLES (Continued).

1. Follow, execute lower back circles with right, 1; back waist circles, arm over front, with left, 2; lower front right, 3; and front waist, arm-over-front, with left, 4. Fig. 18 shows the position of clubs and arms when about to begin this exercise. The broken lines and arrows have nothing to do with this movement. Continue for 24 counts. This is known as the *hip coffee grind, front*.

2. Follow, execute lower back circle with right, 1, back waist circle, arm-over-back, with left, 2; lower front right, 3; and front waist, arm-over-back, with left, 4; make this continuous for 24 counts. Fig. 22 shows the position of clubs and arms when about to begin this movement. The lines and arrows have nothing to do with this exercise, which is known as the *hip coffee grind, back*.

3. Follow, right back waist arm-over-front, 1, lower back left, 2, right front waist, arm over front, 3; lower front left, 4. See Fig. 20 for position of arms and clubs ready to begin. Broken line does not apply to this exercise.

4. Follow, right front waist, arm-over-back circle, 1, left lower front, 2, right back waist, arm-over-

back, 3; left lower back, 4. See Fig. 24 for position of arms and clubs about to begin exercise. Broken lines do not apply.

5. Follow. Practice separately each hand first, then combine. Right lower back, 1, right lower front in median line of body, 3, right back waist arm over front, 5, left back waist, arm over front, 2, lower front in median line of body, 4, and lower back, 6. Fig. 18 shows the clubs and arms in position to begin exercise. The broken line indicates the course taken by the right, and the dotted portions indicate the club's course behind the body. Fig. 20 shows position of arms and clubs just as the lower fronts are completed and the clubs are about to begin the circles behind the body; the broken line shows course taken by right club.

After the exercise has been executed as stated above, either add arm circles or pass them across body with short arm circles (Fig. 21). The broken line indicates direction taken. This exercise, with the Pass, as in Fig. 21, combined with the circles in counts, 1, 2, 3, 4, 5, 6, constitutes what is known as the *lower front fountain.*

6. Follow. Practice separately with each hand, then combine. Right lower front, 1, right lower back in median line of body, 3, right front waist, arm over back, 5, and pass by short arm to right side again, 7; left front waist, arm over back, 2, lower back in median line of body, left lower front, 4, and pass back to

47

position over back, 6. Figures 22, 23, 24, and 25 show the positions of the clubs and arms in executing the various circles. The broken line indicates the course of the right club. The illustrations show how the hands are crossed and recrossed, and how the pass back to starting position is made by short arm. This exercise is known as the *lower back fountain*.

7. Combine the upper fountain with the lower front fountain by executing an extra circle with the right in front of left shoulder. When coming from the lower to the upper fountain execute an extra circle in front of hip with right (front waist right over front).

8. To combine the lower back and lower front fountains. Execute the lower front fountain, and then instead of bringing left over in front bring it over in back, and the arms will be in position to execute the lower back fountain.

To come to the lower front fountain from the lower back after executing the lower back, simply pass left to arm over front instead of arm over back, and proceed with the lower front.

9. Combine upper front fountain with lower front, and run into lower back, then lower front, then lower back, lower front, and up to upper front.

10. Add to exercise 9 follow circles at right and left, also the follow circles directly above head.

11. Execute upper fountain, 1, 2, 3, 4, 5, 6; then bring left under right arm pit, executing an under

arm, 7, while right executes a complete arm circle, 8;
continue the right arm circle, bringing the right under
left arm pit, 10, executing an under arm circle, 12,
while left arm circles out from under right arm pit,
9, and adds a complete arm circle, 11 having thus, for
its counts 7, 9, and 11 executed an under arm circle
and arm circled downward and around to left, upward and across face, and clear around again to position; the right, for 8, 11, and 12, executes one complete arm circle and continues arm-circling until it
reaches the left arm pit, where it executes an under
arm circle.

LESSON V

FOLLOW CIRCLES (Concluded).

1. During the exercise hold the left club horizontal in position occupied by left club in Fig. 16; With the right execute an arm circle, 2, reaching over left wrist, shoulder circle, 4, then, as the club comes out from the shoulder circle, swing under the left club, executing a regular shoulder circle, 6. Counts 4 and 6 are similar to an over arm circle followed immediately by an under arm circle; the left club taking the place of the arm in this case.

2. Hold the right club vertical and about four inches in front of right shoulder, as in the right club position shown in Fig. 16, and maintain this position throughout the entire exercise. Left arm circle, 1; then, as it reaches the position shown in Fig. 16, it reaches forward,—that is, with the backs of the wrists together, the left wrist is extended, thus enabling it to execute a circle in front of the right; the circle is made with the ring grip, 3. (Fig. 12 gives an idea of how the left could reach forward and execute this circle) After having completed this circle the left executes an over arm circle, 5 and is in a position to begin the exercise again.

3. Combine exercises 1 and 2, and what is known as the Tangle will result; this exercise is also known as *twister* and *tying the knot,* each name being quite appropriate.

4. Exercise 3 is sometimes supplemented by the exercise about to be described, the combination being known as the *double tangle;* assuming the description as the supplement, the exercise is begun where exercise 3 is ended. The starting position is then like the position of the arms and clubs in Fig. 16, with the exception that the left is in front of the right. (a) Allow the right club to drop to the horizontal position; both clubs now being parallel, left reaching back executes a circle behind the right shoulder, 7; this circle is practically a left under arm circle, the right club held horizontal representing the arm; as the left club rises while executing the circle just described, begin to extend the wrist, and reaching forward over the right club execute a circle in front of that club, 9. This circle is executed with the ring grip; the left executes an arm circle, 11. (b) Instead of allowing the right to drop horizontal and thereby parallel to the left as in (a), bringing the left vertical and thereby at right angles to the right, extend right wrist, and reaching to right and around under the left club, execute a shoulder circle, 8; still keeping the right wrist over left, execute a circle in front of the left club, 10, and then arm circle, 12.

Combine (a) and (b) and the result will be the

supplement to the tangle; and the two together constitute the double tangle.

5. *Hip tangle.* (a) Starting from position with right, allow left club to hang at arm's length at left side, but about four inches in front of left knee; swing right club by arm-circling, 2, downward and between the left and the knee (see Fig. 20 for position of arms; broken lines do not apply); there, keeping wrists in position, reaching to the right around in front of the left club, execute a circle with the ring grip, 4. (b) Place the right hand on the front of the left hip and point the club obliquely downward left. (Fig. 20 shows the right in practically this position). Now, starting from position with the left, arm-circle downward and execute a lower front in front of the right arm, 1, then, as the lower part of this circle is completed, with the left arm still in front, left wrist on right, and left palm turned backward, reach backward under the right wrist and with the left execute a lower back, behind left hip, 3. Combine the work of right in (a) with the work of left in (b).

6. Execute a lower front fountain, and for the right back waist arm over front, and the left lower back, substitute the hip tangle.

7. With the trunk turned to right, execute forward follow circles continuing these circles as the clubs are gradually brought forward and to the left, the trunk also gradually covering front and then turning left

also; now arm-circle and it will be seen that instead of being a follow right movement it is a follow left.

8. *Over and under.* (a) Hold the left club horizontal and pointing directly forward about a foot in front of the body; with the right, starting from position, execute a forward circle on its own right side, 1; then, reaching over the left club execute a forward circle, this being naturally on the left side of the left arm, 3; just as this circle is completed, lead the club under the left and execute another forward circle, this circle also being on the left side of the left club, 5. (b) Holding the right club horizontal and pointing forward about a foot in front of body, with left starting from position, execute a forward circle 2; reach over right, executing another forward circle, 4; reach under and execute another forward circle, 6. Combine the right hand work of (a) with the left hand work of (b) and the over and under in front of the body is the result.

9. After being able to execute smoothly exercise 8, gradually turning trunk to the right bring the clubs to the right, so that the clubs will be moving in the lateral plane. This exercise thus brought from right to left will change the movement from a follow right to a follow left.

10. Combine upper fountain, double tangle, over and under, lower fountain including hip tangle, and follow circles backward at left.

Based on the material thus far stated, the combinations possible are indefinite in number.

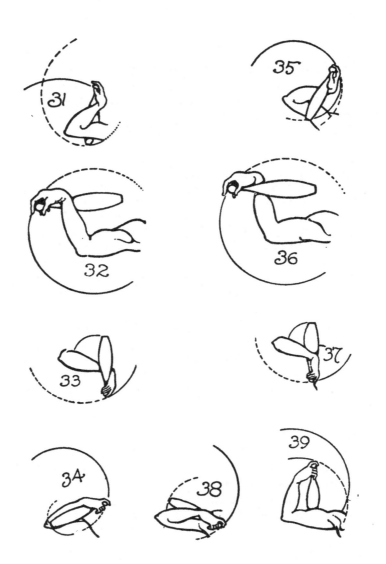

Part III.

ADVANCED CLUB SWINGING, WITH
THE SNAKES.

PART III

ADVANCED CLUB SWINGING, WITH THE SNAKES

The snake movements are considered the most difficult club movements and form the basis of much of the fancy work. These movements are called snakes on account of their fancied resemblance to a snake winding around the arm. There are four principal snakes:

 I. *The outward, or regular snake.*
 II. *The reverse, or inward snake.*
 III. *The forward hip snake.*
 IV. *The reverse, or backward hip snake.*

Combinations of these four with variations and additions form the many kinds of snakes in use. The combinations generally used will be given.

The snakes are all executed with a special *grip,* which is held throughout the entire snake and only released at the *throw off,* the wrist doing the greater part of the work. There are various snake grips used, but the one which seems most satisfactory will be used in the work contained in these lessons and is as follows: The forefinger is placed over the ball or

knob of the club; the other three fingers grasp the
neck or handle; the end of the thumb is placed on the
knob and the ball of the thumb is pressed against the
handle. Figs 34, 48, and 49 give a good idea of the
grip. Another form of the snake grip used is to hold
the club with the thumb and forefinger also on the
neck, so that the club is held with the forefinger and
thumb around the neck, and the ball is on the outside of the ring formed by the thumb and forefinger.

LESSON I

THE OUTWARD SNAKE.

This snake is generally executed in two planes, the horizontal and the vertical; the following description is of the snake executed in the vertical plane. After completing an outward arm circle bend the arm slightly as the club comes over the head and catch the club in the snake grip, holding this grip firmly but not tightly until the throw off; bend the wrist as in Fig. 31, allowing the club to swing behind the arm. The solid line in the illustrations of this snake indicates the course taken by the ends of the club,— either the base, or the handle, or both, as indicated,— to arrive in the position shown in the next illustration. The broken line indicates the course it has taken from the preceding position to arrive at the one shown, and the dotted portions show course of club behind body. (See page 54.)

(a) Bring the base of the club upward, at the same time bringing down the wrist (Figs. 31, 32 and 33), so that the club with the middle point of its long axis as a center, describes a half-circle. Continue the circle, exercising care that the club remains in front of the forearm, and as the hand passes from position shown in Fig. 34 to that in Fig. 35, gradually turn the palm forward, then outward, and the base and handle of the club will describe an entire circle. It will be noticed now that the club, instead of being on the back of the arm, as in Fig. 31, is on the front, and the palm is turned away from the face again.

(b)   Continue the movement as indicated in Figs. 35, 36, 37, 38 and 39, and another circle will have been completed.

(c)   When the club comes to position as in Fig. 39, throw base of club outward and release the snake grip, changing to ordinary grasp; the club will again be ready to proceed with an arm circle. This outward throw with change of grasp is known as the *throw off*.

Summary.   Twice during the snake one could easily touch his nose with his forefinger if he cared to (Figs. 34 and 38).   The first circle starts with the club on the back of the arm (Fig. 31), and the second with the club on the front (Fig. 35); the palm is outward at the beginning of each circle, (a) and (b). There are three distinct efforts, (a), (b), and (c), joined and executed smoothly.   An effort should be made to hold the elbow exactly shoulder high throughout the entire snake, and to bring about the movement of the club by that part of the arm from the elbow down, the main work falling on the wrist. Note how the wrist is worked.   (See page 54.)

In the horizontal snake, as it is generally executed, the club starts as in Fig. 31, but instead of executing its two circles (a) and (b) in the vertical plane, it executes them in the horizontal plane, that is, the club is kept horizontal to the floor during their performance; then, arriving as in Fig. 38, the throw off is executed in the vertical plane again, that is, sideways. The exercises following are executed in the vertical plane from side to side, unless differently stated.

1. Double shoulder snake and double arm circle.

2. Double shoulder snake with upper double fronts.

3. Double shoulder snake, but instead of double arm circle as in exercise 1, throw off and catch the club again, going into another double snake; repeat. This is the *Continuous Snake.*

4. Double shoulder snake, double arm circle, and scissors.

5. Double shoulder snakes and scissors.

6. Double arm circle, double shoulder snakes, double arm circles twice, and double shoulder circle.

7. Alternate movement, shoulder snakes and arm circles; that is, right shoulder snake 1; right arm circle, 2; left arm circle, 1; left shoulder snake, 2.

8. Alternate movement, shoulder snakes and upper fronts.

9. Continuous shoulder snakes; all movements.

10. Same as exercise 9, but occasionally add an arm circle.

LESSON II.

OUTWARD HALF SNAKES.

1. See Lesson I (a). Execute first circle of snake and throw off from position, as in Fig. 34. This is known as the *first half snake.*

2. As in the regular snake, after an arm circle, let the club fall into the snake grip, bending wrist; but in this case allow the club to fall on the front of the arm, Fig. 35, and then execute the second circle of the snake and throw off as in Lesson I, (b) and (c). This is known as the *second half snake.*

3. Double arm circle, double first half snake.

4. Double arm circle, double second half snake.

5. Alternate exercises 3 and 4.

6. Double movement, first half snake; arm circle, second half snake; arm circle and shoulder snake.

These half snakes may be executed horizontally also.

LESSON III.

PERPENDICULAR SNAKE OUTWARD.

Throw into snake grip, as shown in Fig. 31; but instead of making the circle shoulder high, as shown in Figs. 31, 32, 33, and 34, start circling and draw the club downward a little below the waist, circling as shown in Figs. 31, 32, and 33. Its position, instead of being as in Fig. 34, will be as shown in Fig. 54. Next bring the club around back of arm by describing a half circle with its base, handle as center of circle, to position shown in Fig. 53, then to position, shown in Fig. 56; draw the club upward and outward and it will be in position shown in Fig. 38; bring club to position shown in Fig. 39 and throw off. The upward pull is already begun when the club arrives in position shown in Fig. 54. Try to make the club travel up and down in a line perpendicular to the floor.

The exercises of Lesson I apply to this snake also.

LESSON IV.

THE FORWARD HIP SNAKE.

Outward movement from position. (a) Swing the club downward and behind the hip; allow the club to swing as though executing a lower back circle, letting it swing into the snake grip. (Fig. 47 shows the club going behind the hip, and Fig. 40 shows the course, looking from behind, taken by the club to reach the snake grip; and also how the snake grip looks when taken). In the illustrations used to explain the forward hip snake the solid lines indicate the course the club takes to arrive at the next position illustrated; and the broken lines show the course the club has taken from the preceding illustration to arrive at the position held, dotted lines showing the course behind any part of the body.

(b) Fig. 41 shows the club held in the snake grip as seen from the front. Bring it forward (Figs. 42 and 43), keeping it close to the hip, and horizontal to the floor, until it arrives at position shown in Fig. 43. (See page 66.)

(c) Extend the wrist, and let the club move outward and downward (Figs. 43 and 44), and relax the snake grip (Figs. 44 45, and 46) and let the club describe a lower front circle; thus leaving the club ready for another movement.

Practice (a), (b), and (c) until execution is smooth and continuous. In (b) the club is kept close to the body, while (c) is the throw off.

1. *Double hip snake.* In coming forward as in (b), the clubs may either be crossed or held far enough apart so as not to overlap on their upward course; and the same is true in the lower front circle of the throw off. Fig. 59 shows how the clubs in a lower front cross each other.

2. *Double shoulder snake,* throwing off and coming down into double hip snake.

3. *Alternate hip snakes.* These are used more than the double hip snakes.

4. Double hip snake combined with double lower fronts.

5. Combination. With right execute a shoulder snake and with left a hip snake; then with left execute a shoulder snake, and with right a hip snake; continue.

6. Alternate shoulder snakes; follow at once with alternate hip snakes, come up to alternate shoulder snakes, then down to hip snakes, etc. Continue.

7. From position, start double outward arm circle; swing the left behind the body, and with it execute a front waist arm-over-back circle; and having completed this circle, with the left hand still in position behind the body, let the club fall into the snake

grip; then, recrossing the body in back, execute a hip snake, throwing off, coming up to and executing a shoulder circle. Meanwhile the right has completed its arm circle, a shoulder snake, and a shoulder circle.

8. Execute the above with the work of the left given to the right, and the right work given to the left; as in Exercise 7.

9. Combine exercises 7 and 8, omitting the shoulder circles.

10. With one club alone execute a hip snake, but do not throw off. Instead, as club comes to position shown in Fig. 43, let it change slowly to position shown in Fig. 44; then, coming around back of arm until it reaches position shown in Fig. 53, draw the club upward (Fig. 56) until it is on the shoulder (Fig. 38); throw off and catch, executing a shoulder snake.

11. Execute exercise 10, double.

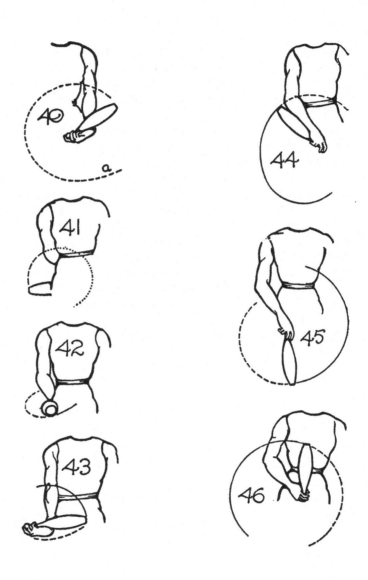

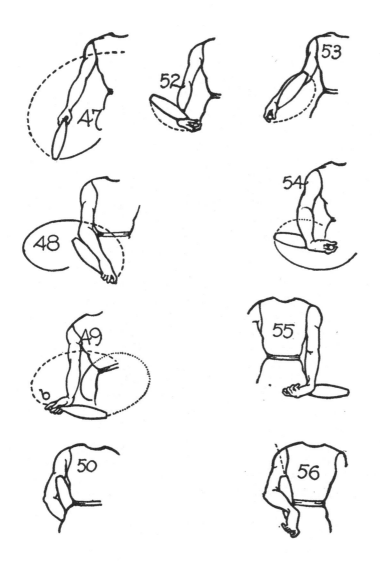

LESSON V.

FORWARD HIP SPIRAL.

Outward Movement: (a) Starting from position shown in Fig. 43, extend the wrist, and the base of the club will follow the course indicated by the solid line. When it arrives at position shown in Fig. 48, the long axis of the club follows course indicated by the solid line, indicating circle. It will be seen that the club has executed a lower front circle, with the club held in the snake grip; the second part is a lower back executed with the snake grip, as follows. (b) Continue the club backward as shown in the dotted and solid line, indicating circle (Fig. 49), describing a circle behind the hip, with club held in snake grip, and coming forward as in Fig. 42, to the position shown in Fig. 43; thus executing the last half of the spiral.

The term *draw spiral* will be used for the following work, first, because of its resemblance to the spiral and because it embraces the draw; secondly, because the use of the term in explaining combinations will help greatly in making matters easily understood. (a) Start a spiral, and as the club comes to position shown in Fig. 49, with the wrist as the center of the half circle to be described, (b), swing the club around outward in front of the arm, in a horizontal plane. (Fig. 52, broken line, shows the course taken by club, and the final position after executing the half circle). (c) Continuous with this half circle draw the club behind the hip, (Fig. 55 shows the draw from behind); continue the circle, the handle leading, backward, outward, and forward in a horizontal plane. (The broken line in Fig. 54 shows the course the club has taken in executing this lower back circle in the horizontal plane with the snake grip and the handle leading). (d) Now, with the wrist as the center of the hand circle to be described, swing the club around in front of the arm, as shown by the solid line in Fig. 54, and the club will be in the starting position, (Fig. 43).

LESSON VI.

TRAVELING SNAKES.

Rope snake. Start regular shoulder snake, and execute the first circle. (The club is now in position shown in Fig. 35). Gradually draw hand downward as the club is executing the work shown in Figs. 35, 36, and 37, and naturally the position instead of being like that shown in Fig. 37 will be as shown in Fig. 50. Continue to draw behind the hip; (Fig. 55 shows how it appears from behind). There it becomes for a while the draw spiral, that is, draw backward and outward, the handle leading, then forward, in a horizontal plane; the broken line of Fig. 54 shows the course the club takes in executing this backward, outward, and forward motion, (horizontal lower back circle), with the handle leading and the long axis of the club following the line described. In Fig. 54, solid line, the club is swung around the front of the arm with the wrist, the center of the half-circle just executed, and the club will be in position shown in Fig. 43. Start to spiral; that is, extend the wrist, (see solid line in Fig. 43), and when the club occupies position shown in Fig. 48 the long axis of the club follows the course indicated by the solid line. Execute thus a lower front circle with the club held in the snake grip and the long axis of the club fol-

70

lowing the circle described. The club will now be in position shown in Fig. 49; the movement becomes a part of the perpendicular snake; that is, draw upward, (Figs. 53, 56) to position shown in Fig. 38, and throw off. The various parts must be joined into one continuous movement, which requires long practice.

1. Double rope snake.

2. Starting simultaneously with both clubs, execute with the right a shoulder snake, and continue to execute rope snakes; with the left start at once continuous rope snakes. In executing the shoulder snake first, and then continuing the rope snakes, it will be seen that as the right starts the first rope snake the left is already executing the draw part of the rope snake; when the right begins to execute the draw part the left will already have completed one rope snake and is beginning a second. Briefly, the right is going down when the left is coming up, and vice-versa. This is the *alternate rope snake.*

3. To get back to the double rope snake, simply add, with either club, a shoulder snake to the rope snake; and the double movement is the result.

4. Rope snake with *roll around head.* Execute rope snake until ready to throw off; but instead of throwing off sweep the club around front of the arm in a half-circle, forward and outward, by turning the palm forward and outward; that is, from position shown in Fig. 39 to position shown in Fig. 31; roll club backward, turning palm up; continue circle in

71

horizontal plane. (In Fig. 57, solid line with arrows shows course club takes). As club is coming forward (solid line in Fig. 58 shows course club takes, and the broken line the space already covered) turn the palm forward and downward; and the club has rolled into the ring grip (Fig. 58). Continuing, the club again arrives at the starting position (Fig. 31). Practice with each hand.

5. Double rope snake with roll around head.

6. Alternate rope snakes with rolls around head.

7. Execute movements shown in Figs. 30, 31, 32, 33, and 34, gradually bringing the hand downward. Start with the movement in Fig. 32; continue the downward motion while executing movements in Figs. 33 and 34; bring club to position shown in Fig. 49, and execute that part of the spiral, the lower back circle with the snake grip (indicated by dotted line in this figure); and as the club comes forward to position shown in Fig. 43, throw off; at the same time drawing the hand upward, throwing the club quickly · into the snake grip above, and executing the first half of the shoulder snake. Throw off and begin movement again. This traveling snake, which is very easy after a little practice, is often substituted for the rope snakes, and is most effective in the double movement. It is known as the counterfeit snake.

8. Execute the double counterfeit snake with roll around head, no throw off above. (See rope snake with roll, exercise 4.)

9. Execute the double counterfeit snake, adding an extra first half snake.

LESSON VII.

THE INWARD SHOULDER SNAKE.

Reverse snake. Execute an inward arm circle, letting club swing inward and downward behind shoulder, as though executing an inward shoulder circle; but catch the club in the snake grip (Fig. 39). The longer solid curve indicates the course followed by the club to reach the position, the broken line indicates the direction the hand is to move to arrive at the next position. The shorter solid line indicates the previous motion of the hand to arrive at this position; the broken line will have the same significance in the following illustrations in regard to the hand and end of the club, and the solid curved line will indicate the direction and course the club and hand have taken to arrive at the position shown. Execute movements as shown in Figs. 38, 37, 36, 35; turn palm forward and inward as the hand travels to position in Fig. 34; proceed as in Figs. 33 and 32. As position in Fig. 31 is taken, extend the wrist and at the same time give a vigorous throw upward, the throw off, and lead club across over head, ready for an arm circle. To summarize, the club executes two circles, inward, and a throw off, and begins each of these circles with the palm turned inward; thus the move-

73

ment as a whole is the reverse, as the name indicates, of the regular shoulder snake.

Inward Movements.

1. Double arm circle and double shoulder snake, continuous.

2. Double upper front and double shoulder snake, then double arm circle, continuous.

3. Double shoulder snake, and, after throw off, catch in snake grip and execute shoulder snake again, continuous.

4. Double shoulder snake, double arm circle, double shoulder circle, arm circle twice, and double shoulder circle, continuous.

The inward shoulder snake executed in the alternate movement does not make as pretty a display as in the double.

5. Alternate movement shoulder snakes and arm circles.

6. Alternate movement shoulder snakes and upper fronts.

7. Continuous alternate shoulder snakes.

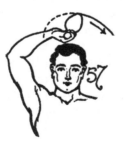 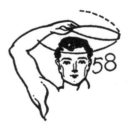

LESSON VIII.

THE REVERSE PERPENDICULAR SNAKE.

Same as the reverse shoulder snake except that the club travels up and down. Start the reverse shoulder snake (Fig. 39), and as the hand and club circle inward, draw the hand down to position shown in Fig. 56 and circle the club around back of arm; Fig. 53 shows how wrist must be slightly extended to allow the club to pass backward (the broken and solid lines having nothing to do with this movement). Continue this movement around back and the club will arrive at position shown in Fig. 54 (the broken and solid lines having nothing to do with this movement). Now continue the motion of the club by circling forward and inward, at the same time drawing the hand upward, and the club will be in position shown in Fig. 33. Continue the movement of the club by assuming position shown in Fig. 32 and throw off directly upward. The club will then be in position for some other movement.

Inward Movements.

1. Double arm circle, double perpendicular snake, continuous.

2. Continuous double perpendicular snake.

3. Double perpendicular snakes, double arm circle, double arm circle twice, double shoulder circle.

75

4. Alternate perpendicular snakes; continuous.

5. Alternate movement, perpendicular snake, and reverse roll around head.

6. Same as exercise 5, but double instead of alternate.

7. Execute a draw spiral (see Lesson VI); and, as club is drawn the second time, instead of continuing draw behind hip, execute the reverse perpendicular snake up the arms and throw off; that is, from the draw position circle the club forward and inward, at the same time drawing club upward to position shown in Fig. 33, then to position shown in Fig. 32, and throw off. This is the reverse rope snake.

8. Execute this exercise in the double movement. Also alternate.

9. To exercise 8, add the reverse roll around head.

10. The inward half snakes are executed similarly to the outward half snakes. For the *inward first half snake* execute the first circle of the inward shoulder snake and throw off.

11. For the *inward second half snake;* from an arm circle throw club into position shown in Fig. 34; that is, allow the club to continue the motion inward from the arm circle as though about to execute an inward hand circle in front of the shoulder, and catching the club in the snake grip, continue the second circle of the shoulder snake and throw off.

12. Double arm circle and double first half snake; continuous.

13. Double arm circle and double second half snake; continuous.

14. Execute exercises 12 and 13 alternately.

15. Double arm circle, double first half snake, double arm circle, double second half snake; double arm circle twice, double shoulder snake, double arm circle and double shoulder circle.

16. Swinging in the outward movement, execute a shoulder circle left and arm circle with the right side to shoulder high at left side, at the same time turning trunk to left; then execute a regular shoulder snake with the left and a reverse with the right, turning trunk from right to left in one continuous movement. Execute a right shoulder circle and a left arm circle to shoulder high at right side; then the right executes a regular shoulder snake and the left a reverse shoulder snake. Repeat the exercise.

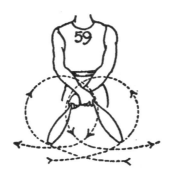

LESSON IX.

INWARD OR REVERSE HIP SNAKE.

The illustrations used for the forward hip snake, if taken in reverse order, with the solid lines used to indicate the course the club has traveled to arrive at the position shown, and the broken line to indicate the course the club is to follow to arrive at the next position, will give the correct result. This snake is, as its name indicates, the reverse of the regular forward snake.

Hold the club as shown in Fig. 46, let it follow the course indicated by the broken line, and it will arrive at position shown in Fig. 45; (see broken line in this and each of the succeeding illustrations). Figs. 44 and 43 show the part of the movement known as *tumbling the club*. Continue as in Fig. 42 and 41 (Fig. 40 shows this position from behind); quickly extend the wrist, or throw off; and the club will take the course shown by the solid line to position shown in Fig. 47; continue movement along the course as shown by the broken line, and the club will have returned to the starting position.

In the tumble the club simply falls downward and at the same time the hand gives a slight jerk upward (Fig. 45), then a little push outward (Fig. 44), so

78

that the force of these combined efforts will tumble the club into position shown in Fig. 43. Care should be exercised that the club is kept close to the body as it travels backward and behind the hip (Figs. 43, 42 and 41). The grip is changed, after the throw off, from the snake grip to the ordinary grasp.

To execute the *double reverse hip snake* in tumbling the clubs, they are crossed in front of the body, and in the throw off they are crossed in back of the body. They can, of course, be held far enough apart so that they do not cross, but the movement is not so pleasing as when they are crossed.

Inward Movements.

1. Double lower front circle and double hip snake, continuous.

2. Add to exercise 1 the double shoulder snake.

3. Alternate hip snakes; these are used more than the double.

4. With the left execute a lower front circle and a hip snake; with the right a shoulder snake and then a shoulder circle; next with the right execute lower front, followed by hip snake, and with the left a shoulder snake and then a shoulder circle.

5. Alternate hip snakes, followed at once with alternate shoulder snakes, continuous.

6. The inward half snakes may be added to the inward movement just as the outward half snakes are combined with the outward movement.

79

7. Catch the club in the snake grip just as if about to execute a regular inward shoulder snake; now sweep the club, with its long axis following the course indicated by the solid line, the handle leading (from 1 to 2, Fig. 68). Continue the sweep as indicated from 2 to 3, where it becomes a regular reverse hip snake, and throw off the club behind the hip. Count slowly; 1, catching the club in the snake grip; 2, as the club sweeps outward; 3, as it passes in front of the hip; and 4, on the throw off. These points are marked in Fig. 68; 4 is executed behind the body. Count slowly, allowing as much time for each count as it takes to execute an entire arm circle. The clubs cross twice in front and once behind the body. If this movement is executed smoothly and correctly it cannot be surpassed for an effective and pleasing movement in fancy club swinging, as the long easy sweep forms a fascinating figure.

8. The regular inward shoulder snake also is executed in the same rhythm as exercise 7, and the circles should be made in long and easy sweeps. In the first circle the club should sweep almost as low as the waist.

LESSON X.

PARALLEL MOVEMENTS.

The movements are all described as going parallel right. It is obvious that the right is working in the outward movement and the left in the inward. The term "parallel" will be used when the movement is parallel from beginning to end; but, for instance, where one club is executing shoulder work and the other lower front work the term "parallel" movements will not be used. The work of each club is designated separately.

1. Parallel shoulder snakes and arm circles.

2. Parallel shoulder snakes and upper fronts.

3. Execute parallel arm circles. After this is completed, the left executes a shoulder snake, while the right executes shoulder circle and arm circle; then the left executes arm circle while the right executes a shoulder snake; then the left executes a shoulder snake while the right executes an arm circle. Continue.

4. Right executes a forward hip snake and a lower front while left executes a lower front and a reverse hip snake. This is the shift (Part II, Lesson II, exercise 11) with the snakes added.

5. Combine parallel shoulder snakes with exercise 4.

6. Parallel shoulder snakes; then turn trunk right and execute parallel circles forward at shoulder height; then, turning front again, execute exercise 4; turn trunk to the left, executing parallel circles backward at shoulder height; turn front again; repeat exercise.

7. Start both clubs from position simultaneously. (a) Left, instead of completing arm circle, executes a front waist arm-over-back; and just as the club comes out from behind the body to the front of the left hip, tumble the club, executing a reverse hip snake; swing up, and execute a shoulder circle. The right, meanwhile, completes its arm circle, executes a shoulder circle, then a shoulder snake, an arm circle, and a shoulder circle. Continue.

8. (b) Left executes arm circle, a shoulder snake, and a shoulder circle, while the right executes a front waist arm-over-back circle, and as the club has completed this circle, it falls into the snake grip behind the body and is brought forward, executing a forward hip snake; it is then thrown off, and coming up, executes a shoulder circle.

9. Combine exercises 7 and 8.

10. To exercise 9, add parallel arm circles, parallel shoulder snake, and parallel arm circles.

11. See Lesson IX, exercise 7. The left executes the same work as in this exercise, while the right starts an outward shoulder snake, and in so doing sweeps around in a circle parallel to that executed by

the left, continuing this parallel movement the right is drawn behind the hip, and executes the lower back circle of the draw spiral. As the club comes to position shown in Fig. 54, the snake grip is relaxed, the club swings downward, and the movement is completed. This movement can be improved if a lower back circle is added to the left and a lower front to the right.

The rhythm is the same in this exercise as in Lesson IX, Exercise 7. Both clubs, after the snake grip is obtained, move with the long axis of the club, handle leading, in the lines they are describing, until they reach the point where the left throws off and the right relaxes its snake grip.

Practice all the above movements parallel left also.

LESSON XI.

REVERSE SPIRAL AND THE FOLLOWS.

Hold the club as in Fig. 49, with the handle leading and the long axis of the club in the circumference of the circle to be described. Follow the course indicated by the broken line, thus executing a lower front circle with the club held in the snake grip. The club, now held as in Fig. 43, travels behind hip (broken lines, Fig. 42), arrives at position shown in Fig. 41, executes a lower back circle, with the club still in the snake grip, and comes to position shown in Fig. 49, ready for another exercise. This is known as the *reverse spiral*.

Follow Movements.

The movements to be described are follows to the right; that is, the right club working in the outward and the left in the inward movement.

1. Follow arm circles and shoulder snakes.
2. Follow shift with snakes added, that is, the left executes lower front and then the reverse hip snake and the right executes a hip snake and lower front afterward.
3. Combine shoulder snakes with exercise 2.
4. See Lesson X, Exercise 6; execute same in follow time.

5. Execute the follow shift, and instead of bringing the left club front leave it behind the body and execute the front waist arm-over-back circle, which is the second circle of the lower back fountain. Continue the lower back fountain.

6. Execute a right lower back, 1, left back waist arm-over-back; 2, lower front right; 3, and left front waist arm-over-back. Substitute the hip snake forward for 1 and 3.

7. Same as exercise 6, but substitute forward hip spirals instead of hip snake.

8. Same as exercise 7, but substitute draw spirals instead of spirals.

9. Same as exercise 6, but after executing the hip snake as stated, execute two spirals and two draw spirals, and continue the circles with the left at the same time.

10. Continuing the circles with the left, as in exercise 6, with the right execute a hip snake, throwing off; and follow it with a shoulder snake, then come down again into a hip snake, etc.

11. Same as exercise 10, continuing circles with left; but with right execute a hip snake, spiral, draw spiral and throw off; run up into shoulder snake and come down again; execute hip snake; then with both execute the lower back fountain. This may be varied by executing the fountain first and then the hip snake, spiral, etc.

12. Lower fountain front, lower back fountain; continue circles with left, then with right hip circle,

draw spiral, throw off and shoulder snake coming down, lower back fountain, etc.

13. Lower back fountain, come back again, and continuing circles with left execute two spirals; then fountain across to left side; and as left club (see Fig. 24) comes to A, tumble it into a reverse spiral, executing two reverse spirals; with the right continue the circles in front and back of left hip.

This *spiral fountain* is especially attractive and pleasing, as, from the front, it looks as though the club were continually spiraling from right to left and left to right.

14. A very pleasing traveling movement and a good way to change from parallel right to parallel left and vice versa. Same as exercise 10; but on coming down, instead of hip snake, with the right pass over and execute front and back waist arm-over-back circles continuously. With the left (see Fig. 22) as the club is coming behind hip, palm turns downward, takes snake grip, and pulls club over to the left; executes forward hip snake, spiral, draw spiral, throwing off and going up to shoulder snake, then comes down again, and both clubs are ready to pass once more to the other side. Continue movement.

15. Follow shoulder snakes; turning trunk to right, follow circles and forward (shoulder) snakes, turning trunk forward, follow shift with snakes added; turning trunk left, backward (reverse) snakes and follow circles; repeat.

This exercise may be executed in the parallel movement also.

Part IV.

EXERCISES FOR CLASS WORK.

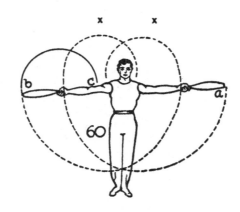

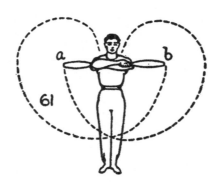

PART IV.

EXERCISES FOR CLASS WORK.

The following exercises, with few exceptions, are modeled mainly like those of Part I, for class work, while those of Parts II and III have been modeled more for individual execution. The former are better for class, the latter for individual, exhibitions.

The exercises of this part, as stated previously, are of the class where the motion of the club is not continuous; that is, where the club is first swung in one direction, then makes a momentary stop and swings in another direction, etc. The following exercises, unlike those given in the other lessons, are executed not only in one vertical plane which corresponds to the lateral plane of the body, but in different vertical planes; that is, planes intersecting the lateral at right and other angles. Exercises executed in the horizontal plane are also included. In addition, the exercises include movements of various parts of the body, such as trunk turning, bending to right and left, stepping and changing, etc.

LESSON I.

CIRCLES.

The *three-quarter-circle* is what its name implies, three-fourths of a circle.

To execute a double inward three-quarter circle,

89

start from position and proceed as though for an inward heart-shaped circle; but when the clubs are rising, after having crossed below, check the motion when the clubs are shoulder high; count 1. (Fig. 60 shows the start and the clubs at shoulder height).

The return from this to the starting position is accomplished by retracing the course just covered; the effort from shoulder high to "x" (Fig. 60) is count 2; and coming down to position from "x" is count 3.

In executing this exercise extend the arms well, reaching out as far as possible, and in completing and beginning another exercise let the movement, (Fig. 60) from "x" to position and back again to "x" be executed with a bound. This bound prepares the way for shoulder circles later on, and is used in ending and beginning all three-quarter-circle exercises.

To execute a double outward three-quarter circle and return to position (see Fig. 61), follow course indicated, clubs shoulder high, elbows also brought up shoulder high, count 1, returning, 2, position, 3.

To execute a three-quarter-parallel-circle and return to position, start from position and proceed as though for the parallel heart-shaped circle, but bring the clubs, in going parallel right, only shoulder high on the left side, 1; and the left will be in position shown as left in Fig. 60, and the right in position shown as right in Fig. 61; returning, 2, position, 3.

1. Double three quarter arm circle outward, 1, returning 2, position, 3.

90

2. Double three quarter arm circle inward, 1, returning, 2, position, 3.

3. Parallel right three quarter arm circle, 1, returning, 2, position, 3. All the parallel movements in this part are described as though starting parallel right.

Tipping or *the slap.* In executing three quarter circles, when the club has risen shoulder high, allow it to swing in a half circle, rest momentarily on the arm, and swing back again. The solid line in Fig. 60 indicates the course followed by the club from "b" to "c" and back again to "b" in executing the slap or tipping. The club in tipping is returned with a bound so that the movement to the arm and back again counts only one.

4. Double three quarter arm circle outward, 1, tipping, 2, returning, 3, position, 4.

5. Same as in exercise 4, but on count 2 quickly bend and straighten the knees (executing a slight squat) to correspond with the time of the tipping.

6. Same as exercise 4, but on 2 add a quick step forward, with right or left, and return. This must be executed with a spring so as to correspond with the tipping.

7. Double three-quarter arm circle inward, 1, with tipping, 2, returning, 3, position, 4.

8. Same leg work as in exercises 5 and 6 may be added to exercise 7.

9. Parallel three-quarter arm circle, 1, tipping, 2, returning, 3, position 4.

10. To exercise 9, add following leg work; on 1, charge the left foot sideways left, returning to position on 3.

11. To exercise 9 add the following leg work; with left foot step sideways left, stride stand, 1, cross right over left in front, cross stand, 2, return to stride stand, 3, position, 4.

12. Same as exercise 11, but instead of crossing right over in front cross it over back of left, 2, and return, 3.

13. Perform alternately exercises 1 and 2; continue to alternate 24 counts.

14. Preform alternately exercises 4 and 7; 24 counts.

15. Perform alternately exercises 5 and 6; 24 counts.

16. Perform alternately exercises 6 and 7; 24 counts.

17. Perform alternately exercise 3, and same exercise parallel left; alternatin gcontinuously 24 counts.

18. Perform alternately exercise 9 and same exercise parallel left; 24 counts.

19. Perform alternately exercise 10 and same exercise parallel left; 24 counts.

20. Perform alternately exercise 11 and same exercise parallel left; 24 counts.

21. Perform alternately exercise 12 and same exercise parallel left; 24 counts.

22. Parallel three quarter circle, turning trunk

left. In this case the right arm remains straight instead of being bent as in exericse 3.

23. Add tipping and leg work to exercise 22; also alternate with same exercise left.

24. Parallel three quarter circle with turning of trunk to left, 1, clubs held firmly (Fig. 62); instead of tipping as in the other exercises, bring the clubs behind the shoulders and return with a snap, 2; returning with trunk turning front, 3; position, 4.

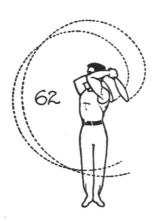

25. Same as exercise 24, but add following leg work; change left foot sideways left, 1, position, 3.

26. Same as exercise 24, with leg work as in exercise 11 and 12.

27. Alternate the same exercise parallel left, with exercises 24, 25, and 26.

28. In the parallel exercises, in alternating with the same exercises, parallel left, as in exercise 17, on count 3, instead of the bound down to position, substitute a hand circle. The exercise will then be:— parallel three quarter arm circle, 1; returning, 2; parallel left shoulder circles, 3; parallel left three quarter arm circles, 4; returning, 5; parallel right shoulder circles, 6; continue 24 counts.

29. Substitute this shoulder circle instead of bound in exercises 17, 18, 19, 20, 21, and 27.

30. Parallel three quarter arm circles, the left executing the three quarter circle in the ordinary way but the right swinging behind the body as in Fig. 63.

31. Same exercise as 30, but change the right foot sideways right and bend body sideways right; this will naturally point the clubs obliquely upward.

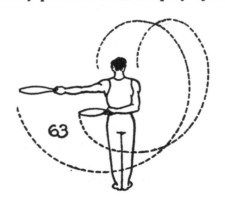

LESSON II.

PENDULUMS.

A pendulum, as the name sugests, is a swinging to and fro, that is, from side to side, and usually from shoulder high to shoulder high, but it may be swung forward and backward, with the arc described more or less than a half circle. A pendulum may be executed with the whole arm or from the elbow down; in fact, any way that brings about a back-and-forth motion.

1. Hold the right club shoulder high, arm extended as in Fig. 60 "b," and the left also at shoulder high (Fig. 61 "a.") Arm circle, 1, that is, execute a pendulum swing from shoulder high at right to shoulder high at left; the right will be as right is shown in Fig. 61 and the left as shown in Fig. 60. Pendulum, i. e., swing back and forth, 1-2, 1-2, 1-2. This is the *parallel pendulum.*

2. Same as exercise 1, with tipping, 1, 2, 3, 4.

3. Same as exercise 2, but add leg work,—side step left on 1, bring right foot to side of left and quickly bend and straighten knees, 2, step to right with right, 3, bring left to side of right and quickly bend and straighten knees, 4.

4. Parallel pendulum from right to left and left

to right as in exercise 1, but turn trunk right. In this movement both arms remain straight throughout entire exercise.

5. Same as exercise 4 with tipping.

6. Parallel pendulum from right to left, 1, execute backward hand circles, 2, pendulum to right, 3, backward hand circles, 4; continue. When the club arrives at left, shoulder high, it is only necessary to allow the club to fall inward toward body as though tipping, but instead continue the hand circle.

These hand circles should be executed first on the outside of the arms and then on the inside (between the arms), continuing to alternate.

7. Same as exercise 6, but execute forward circles on 2 and 4; that is, the club stops at left, shoulder high, executes a forward circle, 2; and same for the other side. Execute circles inside and outside as in exercise 6.

8. Starting at right side as for regular parallel pendulum, the left swings to left, shoulder high, and the right swings behind the body to arm-over-back position (Fig. 63), 1, return, 2.

9. Same as exercise 8, but start with 1 and 2, then pendulum to left side, 3, execute count 1, and 2; but reverse direction for 4 and 5, etc.

10. With right arm extended, shoulder high, left in arm-cross-back position, execute with left a front waist circle, inward movement; and with right hand circle, 1, swing left to left, shoulder high, and right

arm-over-back; execute hand circles, 3, swing to the right, shoulder high with right, and left to arm-over-back; continue.

11. Right extended, shoulder high, left arm-over-back position; with the left execute a front waist circle, 1 (inward movement), swing to left, shoulder high, 2; right swings downward (outward movement) and executes a lower back circle and comes to arm-over-back position, 1, 2. Left swings downward (outward movement), executes a lower back circle, and comes to arm-over-back position, 3, 4, while right executes a front waist (inward movement) and proceeds to shoulder high at right, 3, 4.

12. Hold clubs in position at shoulder high, as shown in Fig. 60 "a" and "b." Pendulum to shoulder high position, as shown in Fig. 61 "a" and "b;" back again, etc.

13. With the right execute three quarter inward arm circle with tipping, 1, 2; same with left, 3, 4; in this exercise the club, instead of bounding back at once, rests on the forearm, 2 and 4; snap the clubs downward off the forearms, in the outward movement (and up to position shown in Fig. 61 "a" and "b"), 5; return inward, double three quarter arm circle, 6, hand circle inward, 7, position, 8.

14. Reverse of above. Three quarter outward right, bringing arm in position shown in Fig. 61 "b," 1, tipping, 2, left three quarter arm circle, 3, tipping, 4; swing from here to the position with arms at sides

shoulder high (Fig. 60 "a" and "b"), 5, double three quarter arm circle, outward movement, 6, outward shoulder circle, 7, position, 8.

15.   Right three quarter arm circle, 1; tip to rest on forearm, 2; right in back, left in front (Fig. 63); left three quarter circle, 3; tip on forearm, 4; swing both clubs to shoulder high at right side, with right in position shown as right in Fig. 60 "b," and left in position shown as left in Fig. 61 "a," 5.   Return with parallel three quarter circle right, 6; parallel shoulder circle right; 7; position, 8.

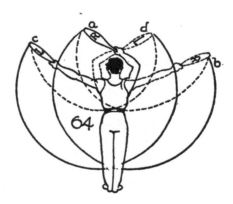

LESSON III.

PENDULUMS (Concluded).

1. With the right execute a bent or short arm swing (Fig. 64 "a" to "b," broken line), 1, swing arm-circle from "b" to "a," solid line, 2; with left arm swing from "c" to "d," (solid line), 1, and execute bent arm swing from "d" to "c," (broken line), 2. In executing the bent arm swings, the club passes behind the head.

2. Execute a bent arm swing from "b" to "a" with right, 1; and arm swing from "a" to "b," 2; with left, arm swing from "d" to "c," 1; and bent arm swing from "c" to "d." This exercise is the reverse of the above.

3. With right club execute an inward arm circle, 1, and proceed as though about to execute a shoulder circle, but as the club comes behind the shoulder reach toward the right so that the club will follow course marked by solid line, Fig. 65; now swing downward from "a" and the club is executing an outward arm circle, 2. This is known as the Pass.

4. With left club execute an outward arm circle, 1, and proceed as though about to execute a shoulder circle, but as the club comes behind the shoulder, pass toward the right so that the club will follow course marked by solid line (Fig. 65). Now

99

swing downward from "b" and the club will execute an inward arm circle, 2.

5. Combine exercises 3 and 4. This method of passing is used generally to come from the parallel left to parallel right, and vice versa.

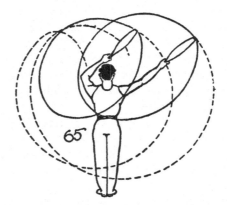

6. Swing double inward arm circle and pass, that is, reach outward after half of the double shoulder circle has been completed; this changes the movement from the double inward to the double outward movement.

7. Change with pass from double outward to double inward.

8. Parallel right, arm circles, 1, pass, 2, to parallel arm circles, left, 3, etc.

9. Parallel right, arm circles, 1, shoulder circles, 2, turning trunk right with forward circles, 3; charge

with right foot to the right and swing the right club
upward, holding it obliquely upward to right, and
swing the left downward till obliquely downward at
left, 4; pass the right club to the left, at same time
swaying to a balance on the left foot, the left knee
bent slightly and the right extended to the right, 5;
parallel arm circles left, and replace right foot, 6;
parallel shoulder circles left, 7; position, 8.

10. Parallel right, arm circles, 1, shoulder circles,
2; with the clubs now in the position shown in Fig.
3, raise the point of the right club so that it will be
vertical, at the same time strike the base of the right
club with the base of the left and simultaneously
charge right foot sideways right, 3; replace foot and
pass the clubs to the left, 4; turning trunk left, execute forward circles, 5; turn front and execute arm
circles, 6, shoulder circles 7, position, 8.

11. Parallel right, arm circles, 1, to shoulder circles, 2; swing left to shoulder high at left side and
swing right to arm-over-back position, 3; coming out,
right executes a lower front and swings up to shoulder high at right side, inward movement, 4 and 5
(the left executes a lower back, outward, going into
an arm-over-back position, 4, 5;) swing both clubs
to left (parallel right movement), 6, shoulder circles,
7, position, 8.

12. Parallel arm circles, 1, shoulder circles, 2;
right executes a shoulder circle and the left a complete arm circle, 3; arm-circle, three quarter, to left

at shoulder high with the left, and the right to arm-over-back position, 4; lower fronts parallel to the left, 5, 6; parallel upper fronts, 7; position, 8.

13. Starting parallel right, three-quarter-circle with left to shoulder high on left side, right to arm-over-back, 1; right lower front, and swing up to right shoulder high, 2, 3, and left lower back circle and to arm-over-back position, 2, 3; left lower front and swing up to left shoulder high, 4, 5, right lower back circle and to arm-over-back position, 4, 5; parallel movement left, arm circles and shoulder circles, 6, 7; position 8.

14. Double outward arm circle and lower front, 1, 2, as arms come to position shown in Fig. 59; raise them to horizontal in front of the body (making the upward movement and completing the lower front in the same motion); now execute the last half of the shoulder snake and throw off, 3, 4; two complete arm circles, 5, 6; shoulder circles, 7; position, 8.

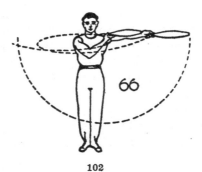

LESSON IV.

COMBINATIONS.

1.   Stand as in Fig. 67, roll the clubs outward, i. e. apart; and, continuing this roll, complete horizontal circle above the arm, 1; pendulum swing to left side, 2; and execute the outward horizontal circles, 3; pendulum to right, 4; etc.

2.   Same as exercise 1, but start the circle by rolling the clubs inward and completing horizontal circles, 1; pendulum, 2, etc.

3.   Hold clubs as in Fig. 66. Roll right club following course indicated by line, thus executing a horizontal circle, with left swing to right as indicated, to position similar to that held by right in the cut; left now executes the horizontal circle and right the pendulum.

4.   Hold clubs as indicated in Fig. 66; execute horizontal circles toward right, with both at same time, and pendulum swing back to position.

5.   Parallel right three quarter circle with turning of trunk left, 1; execute outward horizontal circle, as in exercise 1, 2; returning, 3; position, 4.

6.   Count 1 and 2, as in exercise 5, pendulum to shoulder high right, with trunk turning to right, 3; horizontal circles outward, 4, three quarter circle to position, 5, 6.

103

7. Three quarter parallel right, 1, execute horizontal circles from left to right shoulder high, as in exercise 4, 2; 3; returning, 4; outward shoulder circles, 5; position, 6.

8. Stand as in Fig. 67 and execute horizontal circles above and below the arm, inward; gradually separate hands, bringing left to left side and right to right side. Same exercise with circles outward.

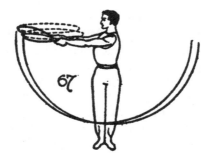

9. The coffee grinder is also executed directly in front of the body. (See explanation on front hip coffee grind, Part II, Lesson IV, Exercise 1.) Swinging clubs thus, bring forward and upward gradually to front and horizontal.

10. In executing the coffee grinder in front of body, introduce snakes; left executing regular snake and right reverse. Use half snakes also.

The tangle and the coffee grinder also combine easily. Coffee grinder is used to pass from one parallel movement to another, i. e., right to left or left to right.

11. A very pretty movement is to execute the coffee grinder horizontally, then gradually bend body forward and bring arms downward, so that the clubs will be executing the movement vertically.

12. Double arm circle and lower front, 1, 2, upper front, 3; charge forward right; and with right arm obliquely forward upward, and left obliquely down backward, allow right club to fall and rest on forearm, 4; bring left club forward upward and swing parallel arm circles to left side, 5; to right side, 6; left side, 7; position, 8.

13. Execute alternate arms and shoulder circle forward.

14. Execute backward circles in same way.

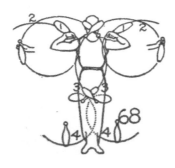

Part V.

GENERAL INFORMATION.

PART V.

GENERAL INFORMATION.

Below are given a few suggestions in the way of executing *facings* while swinging; it is naturally supposed that the pupil is familiar with the regular facings. Care must be observed to keep the clubs moving in the same plane throughout the movements.

1. Execute parallel arm-and-shoulder circle continuously to right, the arm circles being the odd counts, 1, 3, 5, etc., and the shoulder circles the even. On 2 step forward with the left, on 4 pivot on toes, facing about to the right; the clubs preserve the same direction, i. e., if the circles were started toward the right wall of the gymnasium they will still be going that way, but are now parallel circles to the left, as far as the performer is concerned; on 6 the left foot is brought forward to position again; on count 8, instead of executing shoulder circle, come to position. Repeat exercise, starting parallel right again.

2. Going parallel right, swing three quarter arm circle, 1, tip, 2, return, 3, position, 4; as the clubs are being tipped, about face to left, 2; on 4 replace right foot.

Same can be executed substituting forward or backward circles for the tipping, or by omitting these, swinging only the pendulum and facing as the clubs reach shoulder height.

3. Double inward complete arm circle; as the clubs are rising to shoulder height, left about face, i. e., pivot on left heel and support with right toe; now continue the complete arm circle downward and the club is describing a double outward arm circle; execute lower front and come to position, bringing right foot also to position. The double inward circle until the clubs are directly overhead counts 1; as they descend, execute double arm circle, and lower front, count 2 and 3; position, 4; the facing takes place on 2 and the foot is replaced on 4.

4. Double outward movement; swing clubs downward starting arm circles, swing the left behind the body and the right in front of the body, at the same time facing about to left, 1; continue the complete circle overhead and the clubs are now moving inward, 2, execute shoulder circle, also inward, and come to position, i. e., placing foot, on 4.

5. Facing can also be executed in the follow movement while executing forward circles.

Swing a parallel pendulum to left shoulder height, at same time left face; now execute horizontal circles, bringing the arms apart; then proceed with some other exercise.

To *arrange to music* it is best to have the exercise consist of eight counts.

For *torch swinging*, fasten with wire to the end of

an ordinary club a piece of cotton covered with metal gauze, and soak in alcohol; this will serve for ordinary torch swinging. Care must be taken not to have the cotton too wet or the lighted alcohol will fly off when the club is being swung.

As the snake movements are hardly practical for this class of work, the performances should depend on simple circles.

Exhibitions.

For *individual exhibitions of fancy club swinging* use decorated clubs or black clubs with nickeled decorations. Electric lights in or on clubs adapted to the purpose can be used where the current is available.

Below are given suggestions for *class exhibition.* Form the class into four files, with files one and three one step in advance of files two and four.

1. Parallel to right, arm and shoulder circles for 8 counts; same to left; repeat.

2. Double outward arm and shoulder circles, 1, 2, 3, 4, 5, 6; arm circle, 7; position, 8; same exercise, inward movement, 9 to 16; repeat.

3. Parallel to right, three-quarter arm circle with charge to left, i. e., turn trunk to right and execute backward hand circles, 2; return to position by going parallel left, 3 and 4; continue for 16 counts.

4. Double movement, three quarter arm circle outward with tipping and knee bending, 1 and 2, (the arms are crossed in the tipping); return to position, 3

110

and 4; three quarter inward arm circle with tipping, the arms arriving at shoulder height, side horizontal; this with charging obliquely forward left, 5 and 6; return to position, 7 and 8; repeat counts 1, 2, 3, 4, 5, 6, 7, and 8, but the charging takes place obliquely forward right.

Repeat entire exercise, making 32 counts in all.

5. Parallel to left, three quarter arm circles, 1, horizontal circle across front to left shoulder height, (see Lesson IV, Ex. 4), 2 and 3, pendulum back to right shoulder height, 4; repeat counts 2 and 3, repeat count 4, return to position. Repeat entire exercise parallel right. Alternate left and right, 32 counts.

6. Double arm circle outward, 1, double shoulder circle outward, 2, continue through entire exercise 72 counts; 8 counts on place, then files two and four take steps sideways right for 8 counts, while files one and three go sideways left 8 counts; so that files one and two form one file, and files three and four another file; continue the circles 8 counts on place, return to first position in 8 counts, 8 counts on place, then repeat entire process again.

7. Parallel to left, three quarter arm circles, 1; horizontal circles across to left shoulder height, 2 and 3, at same time charging to left; now pendulum right arm to shoulder height right side, left arm swings behind body to arm-over-back, and body is bent sideways left on 4; come to left shoulder

height again with both clubs, 5, tipping, 6, replace left foot and return to position, 7 and 8. Same exercise reversed, 9 to 16. Continue for 32 counts.

8. *a.* Double movement; three quarter arm circle outward with tipping, arms crossed over chest, 1 and 2; let the left come to walk-stand; arm circles inward to shoulder height (arms at side horizontal), with tipping and kneeling on right knee, 3 and 4; return by outward movement to arms crossed, with tipping; at some time raising to feet again, 5 and 6, return to position, 7 and 8. Repeat, coming to right walk stand, kneeling on the left knee.

8. *b.* Parallel left, arm and shoulder circles, 1, 2, 3, 4, 5, 6; arm circle, 7; and position, 8; on count 2 come to right walk stand; on count 4 about face to left by pivoting on toes; remain in this postion, i. e., left walk stand, until count 6; when the foot is replaced. Repeat 8 *a* and 8 *b*.

9. Outward double movement; lower fronts, two shoulder circles, 1, 2, 3, 4; continue for 16 counts. Now execute *b* of exercise 8, then execute the first 16 counts again, and follow by *b* of exercise 8.

10. Inward double arm circle, 1; shoulder circle, 2; arm circle, 3; position, 4; continue for 16 counts. On 2, left toe touch sideways left; on 4, replace; on 6, right toe touch; 8, replace; and so on for 16 counts.

11. Parallel left, arm circles, 1; shoulder circles, 2; turn trunk left and execute forward circles at shoulder height, 3; charge left and swing left club upward

and right downward, halting momentarily with the clubs; now left upward obliquely left and the right obliquely downward right, 4; pass left club behind head and raise right slightly so that they are now again together, at same time that feet are coming back to position again, 5; arm circles parallel right, 6; shoulder circles, 7; position, 8; repeat exercise; continue for 32 counts.

12. Double inward arm and shoulder circles; continue for 8 counts on place; then, as in exercise 6, take 8 side steps forming two files; 8 counts on place, after which the two files thus formed step toward each other, i. e., file one and two as one file step left, and files three and four as one file step right for 8 counts; 8 counts on place come to halt. With clubs on hips files step toward each other, forming twos and march out of gymnasium.

For exhibition by classes of four or eight use a club made of tin, that is, two frustums or cones with their bases soldered together and the handle of a club attached; the effect of these clubs in motion is very dazzling in lamplight, as it gives the appearance of a continuous vibration, and the actual outline of the club is not discernible.

Part VI.

CLUB SWINGING FOR GENERAL AND
CORRECTIVE EXERCISE

PART VI.

CLUB SWINGING FOR GENERAL AND CORRECTIVE EXERCISE.

Club swinging may be made to embrace several substantial general as well as corrective features by emphasizing or exaggerating several details of form. In the case of executing continuous outward double arm circles, the arm is kept fully extended during the entire exercise, and as the clubs come over head, the pupil makes a strong effort to reach as high as possible, as though to touch the ceiling, at the same time raising on the toes; keeping up this stretch as the clubs come through the side horizontal position; and, as the clubs come down, sinking on the heels again. If during the entire exercise a conscious effort is made to keep the chest raised, a strong chest raiser and expander will result. There is a vacuum produced at the apexes of the lungs which is beneficial to the lung proper, while the muscular work, besides being a good shoulder raiser, has a general effect on the external chest as to carriage and make up.

The same is true of the continuous double inward arm circles, except that the stretch sideways takes place as the clubs are coming upward through the side horizontal position and is maintained as the clubs go overhead; then, as the clubs cross and come down, the effort to keep the chest raised must be emphasized.

In executing double outward arm and shoulder circles, the clubs should be raised as high as possible, when the arm circle is started; and on starting the shoulder circle the pupil should make a special effort to draw the elbows back and down, forcibly contracting the muscles between the scalpulas. This makes a good corrective exercise out of a simple movement.

In executing the double inward arm and shoulder circles, the chest is thrown forward by the pupil's special effort, just as the shoulder circles are being made. An attempt should be made to pull the club downward as far behind the shoulders as possible.

The writer has used this method of having the pupil make a special effort at certain points during the execution of the club exercises and results are very encouraging; breathing is usually very much in evidence after several of this class of exercises.

Though suppleness of the wrists is perhaps greatly developed by the snake movements, the deltoid gets the burden of the work, and manifests it unmistakably if this type of movements be executed continuously for a while. Special contraction of muscles between the scapulas as snakes are performed adds to their value.

Change the routine by giving work including lunges, kneeling, and other vigorous leg work, also trunk movements. Marching sideways and execut-

117

ing the class drill given before, with special emphasis on the contraction of the muscles between the shoulders, will make a good combination.

For *endurance* swinging the simple movements are best, such as double inward or outward arm and shoulder circles, adding every now and then a few complete arm circles, changing to the short reel and then the plain follow to the right and left; the reel and the follow movements, from the slight twisting of the body necessary to their execution, exercise a sort of mild massage, said to be very beneficial to the abdomen.

As a form of light work, club swinging stands out as one of the most useful. It satisfies the desire of the pupil to hold or use some sort of apparatus in the performance of exercise. It is, besides, an agreeable change from the ordinary routine light work. There are few forms of exercise which are more pleasing to the eye. No unusual degree of strength is required to take up the work, and, contrary to most forms of exercise, interest for want of variety does not lag as time goes on; but is kept up by the inexhaustible material at hand; and a sort of fascination grows with proficiency.

Rhythm in exercise, upon which so much stress is laid by some writers, is practically coincident with club swinging. Rhythm seems to be a part of the work itself. The work allows easy arrangement into the most attractive and artistic form, developing grace and control of mevement without losing any of its usefulness.

The value of club swinging as a form of exercise is said to have been recognized by the British officers, after England had taken India under its wing; and they forthwith proceeded to annex the new exercise as one of their features of physical training.

A SUGGESTION IN CLUB SWINGING.

By Paul C. Phillips, M. D.

One great obstacle encountered in devising Indian club drills for general exercise has been the difficulty of getting into them sufficient foot-pounds of work to develop organic vigor. The principal measures tried have been the increasing of the weight of the clubs, the use of great circles, and stepping and charging with the feet. All of these, in the experience of most physical directors, have fallen short of producing the desired effect.

Quite recently the writer hit upon the idea of using continuous great circles in combination with lunges to obtain this effect and introduced a series of such movements into a competitive drill. The results were excellent, the whole class puffing at the end of the series, as after the leg work of a Roberts drill.

The series consisted of the following movements, performed with 2 to 3 lb. clubs:

First Half.

1. On count one lunge to right and describe full outside circle to right; on count two return to position and describe another circle like the first. Continue without stopping club for 16 counts.

2. Same as 1 to left side with full left outside circle with left arm and lunge of left leg.

3. On counts one and two as in No. 1; on count three lunge to left, but continue describing full outside circles to right; on four, back to position, describing the same circle; continue without stopping club for 16 counts.

4. Same as No. 3, except that all the circles are to left with the left hand and the first lunge is to left.

5. Full outside circles of both clubs (up cross) with leg work and count as in No. 1.

6. Same circles as in No. 5, with leg work and count as in No. 2.

7. Up cross on count one at R lunge, on two at position, on three at left lunge, on four, at position. Continue without stopping club for 16 counts.

Second Half.

The second half of the series is like the part just given, except that full inside circles are used instead of outside ones.

The above is a simple series, but immediately suggests numerous possibilities for these circles. The foot work may be varied by toe pointing, stepping or charging in different directions, the circles combined in a variety of ways and heavier clubs may be used. The group has intentionally been kept simple, however, to achieve the end aimed at, amount rather than intricacy of work, and the con-

-tinuous full circles and lunges making the best com-bination for its attainment.

The "swing" of these exercises, especially when they are accompanied by the piano, makes them very pleasurable to the gymnast.